Flat Tummy Fix:

The Ultimate Guide to Achieving a Trim and Toned Midsection

BY

Dr. Edna D. Eudy

Copyright © 2023 by Dr. Edna D. Eudy

TABLE OF CONTENT

INTRODUCTION

Vanessa had been struggling with her weight for a while. She had been trying every diet and exercise routine out there to try and get rid of her stubborn belly fat, but nothing seemed to work. She was getting frustrated and starting to give up hope. One day, while browsing the internet, Vanessa came across an article about how certain foods can help you reduce your belly fat. She read the article with great interest and decided to give it a try. The article recommended eating more protein, fiber, and healthy fats. Vanessa started to incorporate these foods into her diet and within a few weeks, she noticed a difference. Her stomach was starting to shrink and her body felt lighter.

She also started to focus more on her exercise routine. She started to do more cardio and strength training exercises to target her stomach area. Vanessa was so excited to see the results of her hard work. After a few months, Vanessa had finally achieved her goal of having a flat stomach. She was so proud of herself for sticking to her plan and not giving up.

Vanessa was now more confident than ever. She no longer felt self-conscious about her body and she was excited to show off her hard work. She was living proof that with dedication and persistence, anything is possible. She was grateful to have found the article that had helped her reach her goals and was happy to share her story with others who were struggling with the same issues. Vanessa was now a positive example of how to achieve a flat stomach and a healthy lifestyle.

Are you tired of struggling to lose weight, despite all your efforts? Have you tried countless diets and exercise programs, only to end up disappointed with the results? If so, the Flat Tummy Fix is the answer you've been searching for. This revolutionary program is designed to help you achieve your desired weight loss goals quickly and effectively. With the Flat Tummy Fix, you'll be able to shed unwanted fat and gain toned, slim muscles in no time. You'll learn how to customize your diet and exercise routine to target stubborn fat deposits, and you'll be able to reach your goals without feeling overwhelmed. So, if you're serious about finally achieving the flat tummy you've always wanted, the Flat Tummy Fix is the perfect solution.

It's time to put an end to your weight loss struggles and finally get the body you've always dreamed of. Get ready to start your journey to a flat tummy with the Flat Tummy Fix.

The Flat Tummy Fix is more than just a diet and exercise program, it's a lifestyle. Get ready to learn how to eat healthier, exercise smarter and make positive changes that will help you reach your goals. With the Flat Tummy Fix, you can finally get the body you've been wanting and the life you deserve. So, let's get started and get that flat tummy you've been dreaming of.

It's time to take the first step towards a healthier, more confident you. With the Flat Tummy Fix, you can finally get the flat tummy you've always wanted. So, let's get started and get that flat tummy you've been dreaming of.

CHAPTER 1
UNDERSTANDING THE BASICS OF FLAT TUMMY FIX

Flat Tummy Fix is an online fitness program created by celebrity trainer Todd Lamb. It is designed to help people lose stubborn belly fat and achieve a toned, flat stomach. The program is based on the combination of three core principles: nutrition, exercise, and lifestyle changes.

The Flat Tummy Fix program includes a 21-day diet plan, an exercise routine, and lifestyle tips to help you get the flat tummy of your dreams. The diet plan focuses on whole foods, healthy fats, and eating in moderation. It also includes recipes for healthy meals and snacks.

The exercise program includes a variety of exercises to help you burn fat, build muscle, and increase your metabolism. It includes both cardio and strength training exercises, and you can choose to do them at home or the gym.

The lifestyle tips are designed to help you stick to the diet and exercise plan and make it into a long-term habit. These tips include stress management techniques, tips on getting enough sleep, and advice on how to stay motivated.

Overall, Flat Tummy Fix is a comprehensive program designed to help you lose belly fat and get a toned, flat stomach. By following the diet, exercise, and lifestyle tips in the program, you can make progress toward your goal.

With the right combination of diet and exercise, you can make a dramatic transformation in your body and reach your fitness goals. So, if you're looking for a way to get a flat stomach, consider giving the Flat Tummy Fix program a try.

Flat Tummy Fix is a comprehensive weight loss program that focuses on helping individuals achieve a flat stomach and overall body transformation. The program is based on a 21-day system that provides a combination of healthy eating habits, exercises, and lifestyle changes that aim to improve your overall health and wellness.

The Flat Tummy Fix program comprises a set of rules and guidelines that help individuals understand the importance of nutrition, hydration, and exercise in achieving a healthy body weight. The program provides detailed information on the types of foods to eat, what to avoid, and the right combination of nutrients to consume to help reduce belly fat.

The program includes a recipe book with delicious and easy-to-prepare meals that help individuals achieve their weight loss goals. The meals are designed to be low in calories, high in nutrients, and with the right balance of macronutrients to promote fat-burning and overall health.

The Flat Tummy Fix program also includes a workout guide with detailed instructions on exercises that help individuals target belly fat, build lean muscle, and improve overall fitness. The workouts are designed to be short, intense, and effective, with a focus on high-intensity interval training (HIIT), which is an effective way to burn fat and improve cardiovascular health.

In addition to nutrition and exercise, the program also emphasizes the importance of lifestyle changes, such as getting enough sleep, managing stress, and staying hydrated. These factors are essential in achieving overall health and wellness and can help individuals maintain their weight loss goals long-term.

Overall, the Flat Tummy Fix program is an effective and comprehensive weight loss program that helps individuals achieve a flat stomach, improve their overall health and wellness, and maintain their weight loss goals long-term. The program is designed to be easy to follow, with detailed instructions and guidelines that make it accessible to individuals of all fitness levels and backgrounds.

The quest for a flat tummy is something that many people desire, but it can be a challenging goal to achieve. However, with the right tools and strategies, it is possible to attain a toned, flat stomach. The Flat Tummy Fix is a weight loss program designed to help individuals achieve their desired body weight and shape, particularly focusing on reducing belly fat. Here is a comprehensive guide to understanding the basics of the Flat Tummy Fix program.

1. **Understanding the Flat Tummy Fix Program:** The Flat Tummy Fix is a 21-day weight loss program designed to help individuals lose weight and achieve a flat stomach. The program comprises a set of rules, guidelines, recipes, and workout plans that promote healthy eating habits, proper hydration, exercise, and lifestyle changes.

2. **How Does Flat Tummy Fix Work?**

The Flat Tummy Fix program works by focusing on three main areas, including nutrition, exercise, and lifestyle changes. The program provides detailed information on the types of foods to eat, the right balance of nutrients, and what to avoid. It also includes a recipe book with easy-to-prepare meals designed to promote fat-burning and overall health.

The program also includes a workout guide with exercises that target belly fat, improve overall fitness, and build lean muscle mass. The workouts are designed to be short, intense, and effective, with a focus on high-intensity interval training (HIIT), which is an effective way to burn fat and improve cardiovascular health.

Additionally, the program emphasizes the importance of lifestyle changes, such as getting enough sleep, managing stress, and staying hydrated. These factors are essential in achieving overall health and wellness and can help individuals maintain their weight loss goals long-term.

3. **Benefits of Flat Tummy Fix:** The benefits of the Flat Tummy Fix program include:

- Reduction in belly fat
- Improved overall health and wellness
- Increased energy levels
- Improved mood and mental clarity
- Better sleep quality

Reduced risk of chronic diseases such as type 2 diabetes, heart disease, and high blood pressure.

4. **Components of the Flat Tummy Fix Program:** The Flat Tummy Fix program comprises several components, including:

- The Flat Tummy Fix Manual: This is a comprehensive guide that provides detailed information on nutrition, exercise, and lifestyle changes to help individuals achieve a flat stomach and overall body transformation.
- The Flat Tummy Fix Recipe Book: This includes a collection of delicious and easy-to-prepare meals that help individuals achieve their weight loss goals. The meals are designed to be low in calories, high in nutrients, and with the right balance of macronutrients to promote fat-burning and overall health.
- The Flat Tummy Fix Workout Guide: This guide provides detailed instructions on exercises that target belly fat, build lean muscle, and improve overall fitness. The workouts are

designed to be short, intense, and effective, with a focus on high-intensity interval training (HIIT).

- The Flat Tummy Fix Video Library: This includes a collection of workout videos that demonstrate the exercises included in the workout guide.

- The Flat Tummy Fix Coaching: This is a support system that provides individuals with guidance, motivation, and accountability to help them stay on track and achieve their weight loss goals.

5. **Who is Flat Tummy Fix Program Suitable For?** The Flat Tummy Fix program is suitable for individuals of all fitness levels and backgrounds who want to achieve a flat stomach and overall body transformation. Whether you are looking to lose a few pounds or want to make a significant change in your body weight and shape, the Flat Tummy Fix program provides a comprehensive approach to weight loss that can help you achieve your goals.

In conclusion, the Flat Tummy Fix program is an effective weight loss program that provides individuals with the tools and strategies they need to do to burn calories.

CHAPTER 2
ASSESSING YOUR CURRENT DIET

Assessing your current diet is a great way to assess your overall health and make sure you're getting the right amount of nutrition. You can do this by keeping a food diary, tracking your intake of essential nutrients, and evaluating the quality of the food you're eating.

First, keeping a food diary is a great way to assess your current diet. Writing down what you eat and when you eat it can help you become more aware of your food choices and patterns. This can help you identify which foods are beneficial for your health and which are not.

Second, tracking your intake of essential nutrients is important. By doing this, you can make sure you're getting the necessary vitamins and minerals your body needs. You can do this by looking up the nutritional information of the food you're eating, or by using a nutrition tracker app.

Finally, evaluating the quality of the food you're eating is important. Eating whole, unprocessed, and nutrient-dense foods is key to good health. It's also important to limit your intake of processed and refined foods, which can be high in sugar, sodium, and unhealthy fats.

By assessing your current diet, you can make sure you're getting the right amount of nutrition and that you're eating a healthy, balanced diet. This can help you maintain good health and improve your overall well-being.

Accessing your current diet is an essential step in achieving your health and wellness goals. Understanding what you eat and how much you eat can help you make informed decisions about your diet and make necessary changes to achieve your desired body weight and shape. Here is a detailed guide on how to access your current diet.

1. Keep a Food Journal:

Keeping a food journal is an effective way to access your current diet. Write down everything you eat and drink for a week, including portion sizes and the time of day, you consumed them. Use a food diary or mobile app to make the process easier.

2. Calculate Your Daily Caloric Intake:

Calculating your daily caloric intake is essential in accessing your current diet. Many online calculators can help you determine the number of calories you need to maintain your current weight. Compare your daily caloric intake to your food journal to determine if you are eating more or less than you should.

3. Determine Your Macronutrient Ratios:

Macronutrients include carbohydrates, proteins, and fats, and are essential for maintaining a healthy diet. Determine your current macronutrient ratios by calculating the percentage of calories you consume from each macronutrient. A balanced diet should consist of approximately 45-65% carbohydrates, 10-35% protein, and 20-35% fat.

4. Evaluate Your Nutrient Intake:

In addition to macronutrients, evaluate your nutrient intake to determine if you are consuming enough vitamins, minerals, and other essential nutrients. Use online resources or consult with a registered dietitian to determine the daily recommended intake for various nutrients and compare them to your food journal.

5. Identify Problem Areas:

Identifying problem areas in your current diet is essential in making necessary changes. Look for patterns in your food journal, such as excessive snacking or high-calorie meals.

Determine areas where you can make changes, such as reducing portion sizes or substituting unhealthy snacks with healthier options.

6. Make Necessary Changes:

After evaluating your current diet, make the necessary changes to achieve your health and wellness goals. Gradual changes are often easier to sustain than drastic changes. Consider making small changes such as reducing portion sizes or substituting unhealthy snacks with healthier options. Also, consider seeking guidance from a registered dietitian or nutritionist to help you develop a sustainable and healthy meal plan.

In conclusion, accessing your current diet is essential in achieving your health and wellness goals. Keeping a food journal, calculating your daily caloric intake, determining your macronutrient ratios, evaluating your nutrient intake, identifying problem areas, and making necessary changes can help you make informed decisions about your diet and achieve your desired body weight and shape. Remember to make gradual changes and seek guidance from a registered dietitian or nutritionist if necessary.

ADDITIONAL BASIC TIPS

1. Keep a food log: Keeping a food log is a great way to track what you eat daily. This can help identify patterns and potential areas for improvement.

2. Know your nutrients: Learning about the different types of nutrients and what they mean for your body is important. Knowing which foods contain the nutrients your body needs can help you make healthier food choices.

3. Talk to a professional: A nutritionist or dietitian can provide helpful advice and feedback on your current diet. They can also help you create a personalized plan to meet your nutrition goals.

4. Pay attention to portion sizes: Eating more food than your body needs can lead to weight gain. Paying attention to portion sizes and being mindful of how much you eat is important for maintaining a healthy diet.

5. Make adjustments: If you find that your diet is lacking in certain areas, make small adjustments to add more nutrients or cut back on unhealthy foods. Making small changes over time can help you make long-term improvements to your diet.

6. Stay hydrated: Staying hydrated is important for overall health. Drinking water throughout the day can help you stay energized and focused.

CHAPTER 3
STRATEGIES FOR EATING HEALTHIER

Eating healthy is an important part of living a healthy and balanced lifestyle. It can be difficult to make changes to your diet, but the benefits are worth it. Making small changes over time can lead to big improvements in your health. This article will provide some strategies for eating healthier that can help you make the transition to a healthier diet.

Some of these strategies include planning out meals in advance, keeping a food journal, reducing or eliminating processed foods, increasing your intake of fruits and vegetables, and increasing your water intake. By following these tips, you will be able to make simple changes to your diet that will have a big impact on your overall health.

Eating healthier is an essential aspect of maintaining a healthy lifestyle. Making healthier food choices can help you achieve your fitness goals, boost your energy levels, and prevent chronic diseases. However, with the abundance of fast food, processed foods, and sugary drinks, it can be challenging to know where to start when it comes to eating healthier. In this context, implementing effective strategies for eating healthier is crucial to ensure that you make sustainable lifestyle changes. This can involve adopting a balanced and nutritious diet, choosing healthier options when dining out and making small but significant changes to your eating habits. By implementing these strategies, you can improve your overall health and well-being, leading to a happier and more fulfilling life.

Eating healthier is an important aspect of maintaining a healthy lifestyle. With so many unhealthy food options available, it can be challenging to choose healthy foods that provide essential nutrients and energy to the body. However, there are several strategies that one can employ to eat healthier and improve their overall health. In this write-up, we will discuss some of these strategies in detail.

- **Plan your meals**: Planning your meals can help you make healthier choices. It enables you to prepare meals that are rich in nutrients and avoid unhealthy options. You can create a weekly meal plan and make a grocery list to ensure that you have all the ingredients you need to prepare healthy meals. This way, you can avoid last-minute unhealthy food choices.

- **Consume a variety of foods**: Eating a variety of foods is essential for a balanced and healthy diet. This includes fruits, vegetables, whole grains, lean proteins, and healthy fats. Consuming a variety of foods ensures that you are getting all the essential nutrients that your body needs to function properly.

- **Control your portion sizes**: Portion control is crucial when it comes to eating healthy. Overeating can lead to weight gain, which can lead to several health problems. By controlling your portion sizes, you can reduce the number of calories you consume and avoid overeating.

- **Avoid processed foods**: Processed foods are often high in calories, sugar, salt, and unhealthy fats. These types of foods can increase your risk of several health problems, such as obesity, high blood pressure, and heart disease. Instead, opt for whole foods that are minimally processed and contain essential nutrients.

- **Drink plenty of water**: Water is essential for the body, and it is essential to drink plenty of water throughout the day.

Water helps to flush out toxins from the body, regulate body temperature, and improve digestion. Aim to drink at least eight glasses of water every day.

- **Limit your intake of sugary drinks and alcohol**: Sugary drinks and alcohol are high in calories and can contribute to weight gain. They can also increase the risk of several health problems, such as diabetes, heart disease, and liver disease. Limit your intake of these drinks to improve your overall health.
- **Cook at home**: Cooking at home enables you to control the ingredients you use, making it easier to prepare healthy meals. It also allows you to experiment with new recipes and flavors and avoid unhealthy food choices.
- **Practice mindful eating**: Mindful eating involves paying attention to the food you eat, how you eat, and the sensations you experience while eating. This can help you to slow down and enjoy your food, which can lead to better digestion and improved overall health.

In conclusion, eating healthier involves making conscious choices about the food you consume. By incorporating these strategies into your daily routine, you can improve your overall health and well-being. Remember, small changes can make a big difference, so start with one or two strategies and gradually incorporate more over time.

IMPORTANCE OF HEALTHY EATING STRATEGIES

Healthy eating strategies are crucial for maintaining good health and preventing chronic diseases. The food we eat provides our bodies with the necessary nutrients and energy to function properly. When we consume unhealthy foods that are high in calories, sugar, salt, and unhealthy fats, it can lead to several health problems, including obesity, high blood pressure, diabetes, and heart disease. Therefore, adopting healthy eating strategies is essential to maintain good health and preventing these health problems.

Here Are Some Reasons Why Healthy Eating Strategies Are Important:

1. **Maintains a healthy weight**: Adopting healthy eating strategies such as portion control, consuming a variety of foods, and avoiding processed foods can help you maintain a healthy weight. Being overweight or obese can increase the risk of several health problems, including heart disease, stroke, diabetes, and certain types of cancer.
2. **Provides essential nutrients**: A healthy diet provides the body with essential nutrients, such as vitamins, minerals, and antioxidants, that are necessary for optimal health. These nutrients play an essential role in maintaining healthy bones, muscles, organs, and overall body function.
3. **Reduces the risk of chronic diseases**: A healthy diet can reduce the risk of chronic diseases, such as heart disease, diabetes, and certain types of cancer. Consuming a diet that is high in fruits, vegetables, whole grains, lean proteins, and healthy fats can help reduce inflammation, control blood sugar levels, and maintain healthy cholesterol levels.
4. **Improves mental health**: Eating a healthy diet can also improve mental health. A diet that is high in fruits, vegetables, and whole grains can improve brain function, memory, and mood. It can also reduce the risk of depression and anxiety.
5. **Boosts energy levels**: Eating a healthy diet can also boost energy levels. Consuming a diet that is rich in whole grains,

lean proteins, and healthy fats can provide the body with sustained energy throughout the day.

CHAPTER 4
EXERCISES TO TONE AND STRENGTHEN YOUR CORE

Core exercises are an important part of any fitness routine. Strengthening your core helps improve balance, posture, and overall stability. Additionally, core exercises can help reduce back pain and prevent injury.

The core muscles are a group of muscles that are responsible for stabilizing the body and providing support for the spine. These muscles are located in the midsection of the body, including the abdomen, lower back, and hips. Strengthening and toning the core muscles is essential for maintaining good posture, preventing back pain, and improving overall body strength. Here are some exercises that can help tone and strengthen your core:

- ❖ **Plank:** The plank is one of the most effective exercises for strengthening the core muscles. To perform the plank, get into a push-up position and lower your body down onto your forearms. Keep your body straight and hold the position for as long as possible.

- ❖ **Crunches**: Crunches are a classic core exercise that can help tone the abdominal muscles. To perform crunches, lie on your back with your knees bent and your hands behind your head. Lift your head, shoulders, and upper back off the ground and hold for a few seconds before lowering back down.

- ❖ **Russian Twist**: The Russian twist is an exercise that targets the oblique muscles. To perform the Russian twist, sit on the ground with your knees bent and your feet flat on the floor. Lean back slightly and lift your feet off the ground. Twist your torso to the right and then to the left, touching your hands to the ground on either side of your body.

❖ **Bicycle Crunch**: The bicycle crunch is another exercise that targets the oblique muscles. To perform the bicycle crunch, lie on your back with your hands behind your head and your knees bent. Lift your head, shoulders, and upper back off the ground and bring your left elbow to your right knee while straightening your left leg. Alternate sides and continue for several reps.

❖ **Side Plank**: The side plank is an exercise that targets the oblique muscles and helps to improve balance. To perform the side plank, lie on your side with your elbow directly under your shoulder and your legs stacked on top of each other. Lift your body off the ground, keeping your body straight, and hold for as long as possible before switching sides.

❖ **Superman**: Superman is an exercise that targets the lower back muscles. To perform the Superman, lie face down on the ground with your arms and legs extended. Lift your arms, legs, and chest off the ground as high as possible and hold for a few seconds before lowering back down.

In conclusion, incorporating these exercises into your workout routine can help to tone and strengthen your core muscles. Remember to start with a few reps and gradually increase the intensity and number of reps over time. Also, be sure to maintain proper form and technique to avoid injury.

13 EXERCISES TO TONE AND STRENGTHEN YOUR CORE

Sure, here are 13 exercises to tone and strengthen your core:

- ❖ **Leg raises**: Lie on your back with your hands under your hips and your legs extended. Lift your legs off the ground and hold for a few seconds before lowering back down.
- ❖ **Scissor kicks**: Lie on your back with your hands under your hips and your legs extended. Lift one leg off the ground and lower the other leg towards the ground. Alternate legs and continue for several reps.
- ❖ **Mountain climbers**: Get into a push-up position and bring your left knee towards your chest. Quickly switch legs and continue for several reps.
- ❖ **Spiderman plank**: Get into a push-up position and bring your left knee towards your left elbow. Switch legs and continue for several reps.
- ❖ **L-sit**: Sit on the ground with your legs extended and your hands by your sides. Lift your body off the ground, keeping your legs straight, and hold for as long as possible.
- ❖ **Reverse crunches**: Lie on your back with your knees bent and your hands behind your head. Lift your legs off the ground and bring your knees towards your chest before lowering back down.
- ❖ **Side crunches**: Lie on your side with your legs stacked on top of each other and your hand behind your head. Lift your upper body off the ground, keeping your body straight, and hold for a few seconds before lowering back down.
- ❖ **Toe touches**: Lie on your back with your legs extended and your arms by your sides. Lift your legs and reach for your toes, holding for a few seconds before lowering back down.
- ❖ **Plank jacks**: Get into a plank position and jump your legs apart and back together.
- ❖ **V-ups**: Lie on your back with your legs and arms extended. Lift your upper body and legs off the ground, bringing

them together in a V-shape, and hold for a few seconds before lowering back down.

- ❖ **Dead bugs**: Lie on your back with your arms extended towards the ceiling and your knees bent. Lower your right arm and left leg towards the ground before switching sides.
- ❖ **Sit-ups**: Lie on your back with your knees bent and your feet flat on the ground. Sit up, bringing your upper body towards your knees before lowering back down.
- ❖ **Woodchoppers**: Stand with your feet shoulder-width apart and hold a weight in your hands. Twist your torso and bring the weight from one side of your body to the other, as if you are chopping wood.

THE NEED TO TRAIN TO TONE AND STRENGTHEN YOUR CORE

Training to tone and strengthen your core is important for a variety of reasons. Firstly, your core muscles, including your abdominals, obliques, and lower back muscles, are responsible for supporting your spine and maintaining good posture. Strengthening these muscles can help prevent back pain and reduce the risk of injury during daily activities or exercise.

In addition, having a strong core can improve athletic performance in many sports, such as running, swimming, and weightlifting. A strong core provides a stable base for movement, allowing for better control and efficiency of movement.

Furthermore, training your core can improve your overall balance and stability. This can be especially beneficial for older adults who may be at a higher risk of falls and injuries.

Lastly, having a toned and strong core can also improve your physical appearance and boost your self-confidence. A defined midsection is often associated with being in good physical shape and can be a source of motivation for maintaining a healthy lifestyle.

IMPORTANCE OF THE ABOVE EXERCISES TO TONE AND STRENGTHEN YOUR CORE

Exercises that tone and strengthen your core are an essential component of any fitness program. A strong core provides a solid foundation for all types of movement, from everyday activities such as sitting and standing, to more complex movements involved in sports and other physical activities. Here are some of the key reasons why exercises that target your core are so important:

- **Improved posture**: Your core muscles help to support your spine and pelvis, which are essential for maintaining good posture. Strengthening these muscles can help improve your overall alignment, reduce the risk of back pain, and improve your ability to sit and stand for long periods.

- **Increased stability and balance**: A strong core provides a stable base for movement, which can help improve your balance and stability. This is especially important as you age, as it can help reduce the risk of falls and other injuries.

- **Enhanced athletic performance**: Many sports and physical activities require a strong and stable core, including running, swimming, and weightlifting. Strengthening your core can improve your ability to generate power, improve your control and efficiency of movement, and reduce the risk of injury during physical activity.

- **Reduced risk of injury**: A strong core can help prevent common injuries, such as lower back pain, by improving the stability of your spine and pelvis. This is especially important for individuals who are engaged in physically demanding activities, such as lifting heavy objects or playing contact sports.
- **Improved appearance**: Toning and strengthening your core can help improve the appearance of your midsection, which can boost your confidence and self-esteem. This is particularly true for individuals who are looking to lose weight or achieve a more defined physique.

In a nutshell, exercises that tone and strengthen your core are essential for overall health and fitness. A strong core can improve your posture, stability, and balance, enhance athletic performance, reduce the risk of injury, and improve your physical appearance. Incorporating core exercises into your fitness routine can help you achieve a well-rounded and effective workout, and ultimately lead to improved health and well-being.

CHAPTER 5
CREATING A CUSTOMIZED WORKOUT ROUTINE

Creating a customized workout routine can be an effective way to achieve your fitness goals, whether you're looking to lose weight, build muscle, or improve your overall health and well-being. Here are some tips for creating a personalized workout routine:

- **Define your goals**: Before creating a workout routine, it's important to define your goals. Are you looking to lose weight, build muscle, or improve your overall fitness? Having a clear idea of what you want to achieve can help guide your workout plan.
- **Assess your fitness level**: Understanding your current fitness level is important for creating a workout plan that is challenging yet achievable. Consider your current fitness level, any physical limitations or injuries, and your overall health.
- **Determine your preferred exercise type**: Consider what types of exercises you enjoy and are willing to do consistently. This could include cardio, strength training, or a combination of both.
- **Decide on the frequency and duration of your workouts**: Determine how often you want to exercise and how long each session will be. This will depend on your schedule and fitness level, but a general guideline is to aim for at least 30 minutes of exercise, 5 days per week.

- **Choose exercises that target your goals**: Select exercises that target the specific goals you identified earlier. For example, if you're looking to build muscle, focus on strength training exercises that target specific muscle groups.

- **Vary your routine:** Mix up your workout routine to keep things interesting and prevent boredom. Incorporate different types of exercises, switch up your routine every few weeks, and challenge yourself with new exercises.
- **Monitor your progress**: Keep track of your progress over time to ensure you're making progress toward your goals. This could include tracking your weight, measuring your body fat percentage, or recording your workout progress.

In summary, creating a customized workout routine involves defining your goals, assessing your fitness level, determining your preferred exercise type, deciding on the frequency and duration of your workouts, choosing exercises that target your goals, varying your routine, and monitoring your progress. By following these steps, you can create an effective workout plan that is tailored to your specific needs and goals.

SCIENTIFIC PROOF FOR CREATING A CUSTOMIZED WORKOUT ROUTINE

Customized workout routines are more effective than generic routines: A study published in the Journal of Strength and Conditioning Research found that participants who followed a customized workout routine based on their fitness level and goals had better results in terms of strength gains and body composition changes compared to those who followed a generic workout plan.

- ✓ **Tailored workout plans can improve adherence**: A study published in the Journal of Sports Science and Medicine found that individuals who received a personalized exercise program were more likely to adhere to the program compared to those who received a generic program.

✓ **Personalized exercise programs can prevent injury**: A study published in the British Journal of Sports Medicine found that personalized exercise programs that took into account an individual's movement patterns and physical limitations were effective in preventing injury.

✓ **Customized programs can improve motivation**: A study published in the Journal of Exercise Science & Fitness found that individuals who followed a personalized exercise program had higher levels of motivation and enjoyment compared to those who followed a generic program.

✓ **Tailored programs can improve overall health**: A review published in the American Journal of Lifestyle Medicine found that personalized exercise programs can lead to improvements in overall health, including reduced risk of chronic diseases such as diabetes, heart disease, and cancer.

RELEVANCE OF WORKOUT PLANS

1. Workout plans help individuals set specific fitness goals and track their progress toward achieving them.
2. They ensure that individuals engage in a balanced exercise routine that targets different muscle groups and fitness components.
3. Following a workout plan helps individuals establish a regular exercise routine, which can improve overall fitness and well-being.
4. A well-designed workout plan can help prevent injury and reduce the risk of developing chronic health conditions.

5. Workout plans can be tailored to an individual's specific fitness level, preferences, and goals, making them more effective and enjoyable.
6. They can provide structure and direction, making it easier for individuals to plan and prioritize their exercise routine amidst a busy lifestyle.
7. Workout plans can also increase motivation by providing a sense of accomplishment as individuals progress toward their fitness goals.

CHAPTER 6
PUTTING IT ALL TOGETHER FOR RESULTS

Putting It All Together for Results in Fixing a flat tummy involves a combination of diet, exercise, and lifestyle changes. A healthy diet is essential for maintaining a flat stomach and should include plenty of fruits, vegetables, whole grains, lean proteins, and healthy fats. Exercise is also important and should involve both cardio and strength training to help burn calories, build muscle, and tone the abdominal muscles. Finally, lifestyle changes such as reducing stress, getting adequate sleep, and avoiding alcohol and processed foods can also help to reduce belly fat. Taking all of these steps together can help you achieve a flat stomach in no time.

In terms of diet, focus on eating small, frequent meals throughout the day, containing a balanced mix of macronutrients. Try to include a variety of colorful fruits and vegetables, lean proteins, whole grains, and healthy fats in your meals. Avoid highly processed foods such as white bread, white pasta, and sugary snacks, and limit your intake of alcohol.

In terms of exercise, aim to do both cardio and strength training exercises. Cardio exercises such as jogging, cycling, and swimming can help to burn calories and fat, while strength training can help to build muscle, tone the abdominal muscles, and strengthen the core. Aim for at least 30 minutes of exercise a day, and don't forget to add in some stretching exercises too.

Finally, lifestyle changes can also help to reduce belly fat. Try to reduce stress levels by taking regular breaks, getting enough sleep, and practicing relaxation techniques such as yoga or meditation. Avoiding alcohol and processed foods is also important, as these can contribute to an increased waistline. By taking all of these steps together, you can help to reduce belly fat and achieve a flatter stomach. Remember, it takes time and consistency to see results, so stick with it and be patient. With dedication and hard work, you will be well on your way to achieving a flat tummy in no time.

Achieving a flat belly requires a combination of factors, including exercise, diet, and lifestyle changes. Here are some notes on how to put it all together for effective results in fixing a flat belly:

- o **Exercise**: One of the most effective ways to reduce belly fat is through exercise. Focus on exercises that target the core muscles such as crunches, planks, and bicycle crunches. Aim for at least 30 minutes of moderate-intensity exercise five days a week. Mix it up with cardio exercises such as running, cycling, or swimming to burn calories and reduce overall body fat.
- o **Diet**: What you eat plays a significant role in reducing belly fat. To achieve a flat belly, aim for a balanced diet that includes lean protein, healthy fats, and complex carbohydrates. Avoid sugary and processed foods, which can contribute to belly fat. Increase your intake of fruits, vegetables, and whole grains, which are rich in fiber and can help you feel fuller for longer.
- o **Hydration**: Staying hydrated is essential for good health and can also help you achieve a flat belly. Drinking plenty of water helps flush out toxins and reduce bloating. Aim for at least 8-10 glasses of water a day, and avoid sugary drinks, which can contribute to belly fat.

- o **Sleep:** Getting enough sleep is crucial for good health, including maintaining a flat belly. Lack of sleep can lead to weight gain and increased belly fat. Aim for at least 7-8 hours of sleep each night, and try to maintain a regular sleep schedule.
- o **Stress management**: Chronic stress can lead to increased levels of cortisol, a hormone that can contribute to belly fat. Finding ways to manage stress, such as meditation, yoga, or deep breathing, can help reduce cortisol levels and promote a flat belly.

In conclusion, achieving a flat belly requires a comprehensive approach that includes exercise, diet, hydration, sleep, and stress management. By incorporating these elements into your daily routine, you can achieve your goal of a flat belly and improved overall health.

SIGNS OF A REDUCED BELLY

Reducing belly fat has many health benefits, and several signs and symptoms indicate you have successfully reduced your belly fat. Here are some signs and symptoms of a reduced belly:

1. **Smaller waist circumference**: A smaller waist circumference is a clear indication of reduced belly fat. If you notice that your waistline is smaller than it was before, it is a sign that you have successfully reduced belly fat.
2. **Improved body composition**: A reduced belly is a sign that you have improved your body composition. With less belly fat, you will have more muscle mass and less body fat, which can improve your overall health and fitness.
3. **Improved physical performance**: As you reduce belly fat, you may find that your physical performance improves.

You may be able to perform physical activities with greater ease, and you may feel more energized during exercise.

4. **Reduced risk of chronic diseases**: Belly fat is associated with an increased risk of chronic diseases such as type 2 diabetes, heart disease, and stroke. With a reduced belly, you are likely to have a lower risk of developing these conditions.

5. **Reduced inflammation**: Excess belly fat is associated with increased inflammation in the body. With a reduced belly, you may notice a reduction in inflammation, which can improve your overall health and reduce your risk of chronic diseases.

6. **Improved digestion**: Excess belly fat can contribute to digestive issues such as bloating, constipation, and acid reflux. With a reduced belly, you may find that your digestion improves, and you experience fewer digestive symptoms.

CONCLUSION

The Flat Tummy Fix is a powerful program that can help you achieve your weight-loss goals. Its combination of effective nutrition, exercise, and lifestyle changes is designed to help you achieve the best results. It's important to remember that this program isn't a magical cure-all and that it requires commitment and dedication. With that said, the Flat Tummy Fix is an effective way to reach your goals and can be a great way to kick-start your weight-loss journey. With the right mindset and dedication, you can reach your goals and feel great about yourself.

The key takeaway is that the Flat Tummy Fix is a powerful program that can help you reach your weight-loss goals with dedication and commitment. With the right attitude, you can be successful in the program and feel great about yourself. There are no shortcuts to weight loss and it takes time, but with the Flat Tummy Fix, you can get closer to your goals and feel great about yourself in the process.

So, if you're ready to take the first step and make a commitment to yourself, the Flat Tummy Fix is a great way to start your journey. With the right mindset and dedication, you can reach your goals and feel great about yourself.

The Flat Tummy Fix is a comprehensive weight loss program designed to help people lose weight and achieve a slimmer, more toned physique. This program offers a variety of tools and resources to help you achieve your weight loss goals, including meal plans, workout routines, and a supportive community of like-minded individuals. But the real power of the Flat Tummy Fix lies in its ability to transform your mindset and help you develop a sustainable, healthy lifestyle that will last long after you've reached your ideal weight.

At the heart of the Flat Tummy Fix is a commitment to holistic wellness. This program recognizes that weight loss is about more than just shedding pounds; it's about improving your overall health and well-being. That's why the Flat Tummy Fix focuses on helping you develop healthy habits that will support your weight loss journey and improve your quality of life.

One of the key components of the Flat Tummy Fix is its emphasis on whole, nutritious foods. The program's meal plans are designed to provide you with a balanced, healthy diet that will fuel your body and help you achieve optimal health. By eating a variety of fruits, vegetables, lean proteins, and healthy fats, you'll be able to nourish your body and support your weight loss goals at the same time.

But the Flat Tummy Fix doesn't just focus on what you eat; it also emphasizes the importance of physical activity. The program includes a variety of workout routines designed to help you burn fat, tone your muscles, and improve your overall fitness level. Whether you prefer high-intensity interval training or gentle yoga, there's a workout routine in the Flat Tummy Fix that will meet your needs.

Perhaps one of the most powerful aspects of the Flat Tummy Fix is its community of supportive individuals. When you join the program, you'll be connected with like-minded people who are also on a weight loss journey. This community provides a source of encouragement and motivation, helping you stay on track and achieve your goals.

But the true power of the Flat Tummy Fix lies in its ability to transform your mindset. This program is not just about losing weight; it's about developing a healthy relationship with food, exercise, and your body. By learning to appreciate your body and treat it with kindness and respect, you'll be able to create lasting change and maintain a healthy weight for life.

So how does the Flat Tummy Fix help you transform your mindset? One way is by focusing on the power of positive thinking. This program encourages you to adopt a positive, can-do attitude and believes in yourself and your ability to succeed. By focusing on your strengths and successes, rather than your failures and setbacks, you'll be able to build confidence and stay motivated.

Another way the Flat Tummy Fix helps you transform your mindset is by encouraging you to develop a growth mindset. This means embracing challenges and viewing them as opportunities for learning and growth. Rather than giving up when you encounter obstacles, you'll be able to see them as opportunities to develop new skills and improve your abilities. Finally, the Flat Tummy Fix helps you transform your mindset by teaching you to focus on the present moment. Rather than dwelling on past mistakes or worrying about the future, this program encourages you to be present in the here and now. By focusing on the present moment and making healthy choices in the here and now, you'll be able to create a better future for yourself.

In conclusion, the Flat Tummy Fix is a powerful weight loss program that can help you achieve your goals and transform your life. Whether you're looking to lose a few pounds or make a complete lifestyle change, this program can help you develop healthy habits that will support your weight loss journey and improve your overall well-being. By embracing a positive, growth-focused mindset and staying committed to your goals, you'll be able to achieve lasting success.